Witches, Midwives, and Nurses
A History of Women Healers

by Barbara Ehrenreich
and Deirdre English

The Feminist Press
at The City University of New York
New York

Published in the United States by The Feminist Press at the City University of New York, City College/CUNY, Wingate Hall, Convent Avenue at 138 Street, New York, NY 10031

ISBN 0-912670-13-4

Printed in Canada by Webcom Limited

03 02 01 00 99 98 25 24 23 22 21 20 19 18

Introduction

Women have always been healers. They were the unlicensed doctors and anatomists of western history. They were abortionists, nurses and counsellors. They were pharmacists, cultivating healing herbs and exchanging the secrets of their uses. They were midwives, travelling from home to home and village to village. For centuries women were doctors without degrees, barred from books and lectures, learning from each other, and passing on experience from neighbor to neighbor and mother to daughter. They were called "wise women" by the people, witches or charlatans by the authorities. Medicine is part of our heritage as women, our history, our birthright.

Today, however, health care is the property of male professionals. Ninety-three percent of the doctors in the US are men; and almost all the top directors and administrators of health institutions. Women are still in the overall majority—70 percent of health workers are women—but we have been incorporated as *workers* into an industry where the bosses are men. We are no longer independent practitioners, known by our own names, for our own work. We are, for the most part, institutional fixtures, filling faceless job slots: clerk, dietary aide, technician, maid.

When we are allowed to participate in the healing process, we can do so only nurses. And nurses of every rank from aide up are just "ancillary workers" in relation to the doctors (from the Latin *ancilla*, maid servant). From the nurses' aide, whose menial tasks are spelled out with industrial precision, to the "professional" nurse, who translates the doctors' orders into the aide's tasks, nurses share the status of a uniformed maid service to the dominant male professionals.

Our subservience is reinforced by our ignorance, and our ignorance is *enforced*. Nurses are taught not to question, not to challenge. "The doctor knows best." He is the shaman, in touch with the forbidden, mystically complex world of Science which we have been taught is beyond our grasp. Women health workers are alienated from the scientific substance of their work, restricted to the "womanly" business of nurturing and housekeeping—a passive, silent majority.

We are told that our subservience is biologically ordained: women are inherently nurse-like and not doctor-like. Sometimes we even try to console ourselves with the theory that we *were* defeated by anatomy before we were defeated by men, that women have been so trapped by the cycles of menstruation and reproduction that they have never been free and creative agents outside their homes. Another myth, fostered by conventional medical histories, is that male professionals won out on the strength of their superior technology. According to these accounts, (male) science more or less automatically replaced (female) superstition—which from then on was called "old wives' tales."

But history belies these theories. Women have been autonomous healers, often the only healers for women and the poor. And we found, in the periods we have studied, that, if anything, it was the male professionals who clung to untested doctrines and ritualistic practices—and it was the women healers who represented a more humane, empirical approach to healing.

Our position in the health system today is not "natural." It is a condition which has to be explained. In this pamphlet we have asked: How did we arrive at our present position of subservience from our former position of leadership?

We learned this much: That the suppression of women health workers and the rise to dominance of male professionals was not a "natural" process, resulting automatically from changes in medical science, nor was it the result of women's failure to take on healing work. It was an active *takeover* by male professionals. And it was not science that enabled men to win out: The critical battles took place long before the development of modern scientific technology.

The stakes of the struggle were high: Political and economic monopolization of medicine meant control over its institutional organizations, its theory and practice, its profits and prestige. And the stakes are even higher today, when total control of medicine means potential power to determine who will live and will die, who is fertile and who is sterile, who is "mad" and who sane.

The suppression of female healers by the medical establishment was a political struggle, first, in that it is part of the history of sex struggle in general. The status of women healers has risen and fallen with the status of women When women healers were attacked, they were attacked *as Women*; when they fought back, they fought back in solidarity with all women.

It was a political struggle, second, in that it was part of a *class* struggle. Women healers were people's doctors, and their medicine was part of a people's subculture. To this very day women's medical practice has thrived in the midst of rebellious lower class movements which have struggled to be free from the established authorities. Male professionals, on the other hand, served the ruling class — both medically and politically. Their interests have been advanced by the universities, the philanthropic foundations and the law. They owe their victory — not so much to their own efforts — but to the intervention of the ruling class they served.

This pamphlet represents a beginning of the research which will have to be done to recapture our history as health workers. It is a fragmentary account, assembled from sources which were usually sketchy and often biased, by women who are in no sense "professional" historians. We confined ourselves to western history, since the institutions we confront today are the products of western civilization. We are far from being able to present a complete chronological history. Instead, we looked at two separate, important phases in the male takeover of health care: the suppression of witches in medieval Europe, and the rise of the male medical profession in 19th century America.

To know our history is to begin to see how to take up the struggle again.

Witchcraft and Medicine in the Middle Ages

Witches lived and were burned long before the development of modern medical technology. The great majority of them were lay healers serving the peasant population, and their suppression marks one of the opening struggles in the history of man's suppression of women as healers.

The other side of the suppression of witches as healers was the creation of a new male medical profession, under the protection and patronage of the ruling classes. This new European medical profession played an important role in the witch-hunts, supporting the witches' persecutors with "medical" reasoning:

> . . . . Because the Medieval Church, with the support of kings, princes and secular authorities, controlled medical education and practice, the Inquisition [witch-hunts] constitutes, among other things, an early instance of the "professional" repudiating the skills and interfering with the rights of the "nonprofessional" to minister to the poor. (Thomas Szasz, *The Manufacture of Madness*)

The witch-hunts left a lasting effect: An aspect of the female has ever since been associated with the witch, and an aura of contamination has remained—especially around the midwife and other women healers. This early and devastating exclusion of women from independent healing roles was a violent precedent and a warning: It was to become a theme of our history. The women's health movement of today has ancient roots in the medieval covens, and its opponents have as their ancestors those who ruthlessly forced the elimination of witches.

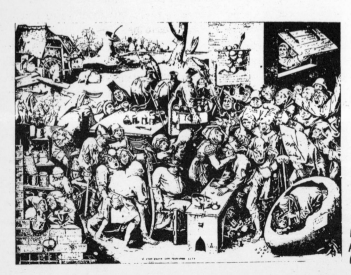

Witch healing peasants (Brueghel)

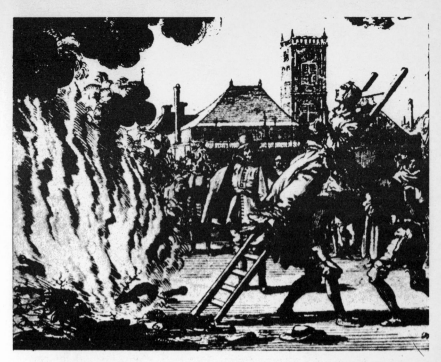

The Witch Craze

The age of witch-hunting spanned more than four centuries (from the 14th to the 17th century) in its sweep from Germany to England. It was born in feudalism and lasted — gaining in virulence — well into the "age of reason." The witch-craze took different forms at different times and places, but never lost its essential character: that of a ruling class campaign of terror directed against the female peasant population. Witches represented a political, religious and sexual threat to the Protestant and Catholic churches alike, as well as to the state.

The extent of the witch-craze is startling: In the late fifteenth and early sixteenth centuries there were thousands upon thousands of executions — usually live burnings at the stake — in Germany, Italy and other countries. In the mid-sixteenth century the terror spread to France, and finally to England. One writer has estimated the number of executions at an average of 600 a year for certain German cities — or two a day, "leaving out Sundays". Nine-hundred witches were destroyed in a single year in the Wertzberg area, and 1000 in and around Como. At Toulouse, four-hundred were put to death in a day. In the Bishopric of Trier, in 1585, two villages were left with only one female inhabitant each. Many writers have estimated the total number killed to have been in the

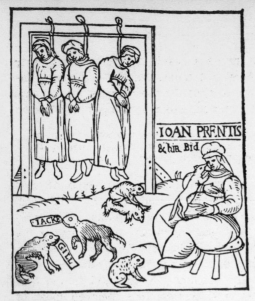

Three witches hanging, from the title page of a contemporary pamphlet on the third Chelmsford witch trial, 1589

millions. Women made up some 85 percent of those executed—old women, young women and children. *

Their scope alone suggests that the witch hunts represent a deep-seated social phenomenon which goes far beyond the history of medicine. In locale and timing, the most virulent witch hunts were associated with periods of great social upheaval shaking feudalism at its roots—mass peasant uprisings and conspiracies, the beginnings of capitalism, and the rise of Protestantism. There is fragmentary evidence—which feminists ought to follow up—suggesting that in some areas witchcraft represented a female-led peasant rebellion. Here we can't attempt to explore the historical context of the witch hunts in any depth. But we do have to get beyond some common myths about the witch-craze—myths which rob the "witch" of any dignity and put the blame on her and the peasants she served.

Unfortunately, the witch herself—poor and illiterate—did not leave us her story. It was recorded, like all history, by the educated elite, so that today we know the witch only through the eyes of her persecutors.

Two of the most common theories of the witch hunts are basically *medical* interpretations, attributing the witch craze to unexplainable outbreaks of mass hysteria. One version has it that the peasantry went mad. According to this, the witch-craze was an

---

* We are omitting from this discussion any mention of the New England witch trials in the 1600's. These trials occurred on a relatively small scale, very late in the history of witch-hunts, and in an entirely different social context than the earlier European witch-craze.

epidemic of mass hatred and panic cast in images of a blood-lusty peasant mob bearing flaming torches. Another psychiatric interpretation holds that the witches themselves were insane. One authoritative psychiatric historian, Gregory Zilboorg, wrote that:

> ...millions of witches, sorcerers, possessed and obsessed were an enormous mass of severe neurotics [and] psychotics...for many years the world looked like a veritable insane asylum...

But, in fact, the witch-craze was neither a lynching party nor a mass suicide by hysterical women. Rather, it followed well-ordered, legalistic procedures. The witch-hunts were well-organized campaigns, initiated, financed and executed by Church and State. To Catholic and Protestant witch-hunters alike, the unquestioned authority on how to conduct a witch hunt was the *Malleus Maleficarum*, or *Hammer of Witches*, written in 1484 by the Reverends Kramer and Sprenger (the "beloved sons" of Pope Innocent VIII.) For three centuries this sadistic book lay on the bench of every judge, every witch-hunter. In a long section on judicial proceedings, the instructions make it clear how the "hysteria" was set off:

The job of initiating a witch trial was to be performed by either the Vicar (priest) or Judge of the County, who was to post a notice to

> direct, command, require and admonish that within the space of twelve days...that they should reveal it unto us if anyone know, see or have heard that any person is reported to be a heretic or a witch, or if any is suspected especially of such practices as cause injury to men, cattle, or the fruits of the earth, to the loss of the State.

Anyone failing to report a witch faced both excommunication and a long list of temporal punishments.

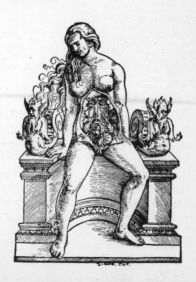

If this threatening notice exposed at least one witch, her trial could be used to unearth several more. Kramer and Sprenger gave detailed instructions about the use of tortures to force confessions and further accusations. Commonly, the accused was stripped naked and shaved of all her body hair, then subjected to thumb-screws and the rack, spikes and bone-crushing "boots," starvation and beatings. The point is obvious: The witch-craze did not arise spontaneously in the peasantry. It was a calculated ruling class campaign of terrorization.

The Crimes of the Witches

Who were the witches, then, and what were their "crimes" that could arouse such vicious upper class suppression? Undoubtedly, over the centuries of witch hunting, the charge of "witchcraft" came to cover a multitude of sins ranging from political subversion and religious heresy to lewdness and blasphemy. But three central accusations emerge repeatedly in the history of witchcraft throughout northern Europe: First, witches are accused of every conceivable sexual crime against men. Quite simply, they are "accused" of female sexuality. Second, they are accused of being organized. Third, they are accused of having magical powers affecting health—of harming, but also of healing. They were often charged specifically with possessing medical and obstetrical skills.

First, consider the charge of sexual crimes. The medieval Catholic Church elevated sexism to a point of principle: The *Malleus* declares, "When a woman thinks alone, she thinks evil." The misogyny of the Church, if not proved by the witch-craze itself, is demonstrated by its teaching that in intercourse the male deposits in the female a homunculus, or "little person," complete

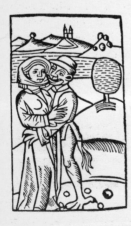

Devil seducing a witch

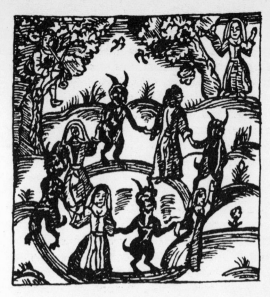

Witches and demons dancing in a ring

with soul, which is simply housed in the womb for nine months, without acquiring any attributes of the mother. The homunculus is not really safe, however, until it reaches male hands again, when a priest baptises it, ensuring the salvation of its immortal soul.

Another depressing fantasy of some medieval religious thinkers was that upon resurrection all human beings would be reborn as men!

The Church associated women with sex, and all pleasure in sex was condemned, because it could only come from the devil. Witches were supposed to have gotten pleasure from copulation with the devil (despite the icy-cold organ he was reputed to possess) and they in turn infected men. Lust in either man or wife, then, was blamed on the female. On the other hand, witches were accused of making men impotent and of causing their penises to disappear. As for female sexuality, witches were accused, in effect, of giving contraceptive aid and of performing abortions:

Now there are, as it is said in the Papal Bull, seven methods by which they infect with witchcraft the venereal act and the conception of the womb: First, by inclining the minds of men to inordinate passion; second, by obstructing their generative force; third, by removing the members accommodated to that act; fourth, by changing men into beasts by their magic act; fifth, by destroying the generative force in women; sixth, by procuring abortion; seventh, by offering children to the devils, besides other animals and fruits of the earth with which they work much harm...

(*Malleus Maleficarum*)

In the eyes of the Church, all the witches' power was ultimately derived from her sexuality. Her career began with sexual intercourse with the devil. Each witch was confirmed at a general meeting (the witches' Sabbath) at which the devil presided, often in the form of a goat, and had intercourse with the neophytes. In return for her powers, the witch promised to serve him faithfully. (In the imagination of the Church even evil could only be thought of as ultimately male-directed!) As the *Malleus* makes clear, the devil almost always acts through the female, just as he did in Eden:

All witchcraft comes from carnal lust, which in women is insatiable...Wherefore for the sake of fulfilling their lusts they consort with devils...it is sufficiently clear that it is no matter for wonder that there are more women than men found infected with the heresy of witchcraft...And blessed be the Highest Who has so far preserved the male sex from so great a crime...

Not only were the witches women—they were women who seemed to be organized into an enormous secret society. A witch who was a proved member of the "Devil's party" was more dreadful than one who had acted alone, and the witch-hunting literature is obsessed with the question of what went on at the witches' "Sabbaths." (Eating of unbaptised babies? Bestialism and mass orgies? So went their lurid speculations...)

In fact, there is evidence that women accused of being witches did meet locally in small groups and that these groups came together in crowds of hundreds or thousands on festival days. Some writers speculate that the meetings were occasions for pagan religious worship. Undoubtedly the meetings were also occasions for trading herbal lore and passing on the news. We have little evidence about the political significance of the witches' organizations, but it's hard to imagine that they weren't connected to the peasant rebellions of the time. Any peasant organization, just by being an organization, would attract dissidents, increase communication between villages, and build a spirit of collectivity and autonomy among the peasants.

Witches as Healers

We come now to the most fantastic accusation of all: The witch is accused not only of murdering and poisoning, sex crimes and conspiracy—but of *helping and healing*. As a leading English witch-hunter put it:

For this must always be remembered, as a conclusion, that by witches we understand not only those which kill and torment, but all Diviners, Charmers, Jugglers, all Wizards, commonly called wise men and wise women...and in the same number we reckon all good Witches, which

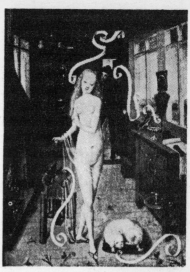

Witch preparing a potion

do no hurt but good, which do not spoil and destroy, but save and deliver...It were a thousand times better for the land if all Witches, but especially the blessing Witch, might suffer death.

Witch-healers were often the only general medical practitioners for a people who had no doctors and no hospitals and who were bitterly afflicted with poverty and disease. In particular, the association of the witch and the midwife was strong: "No one does more harm to the Catholic Church than midwives," wrote witch-hunters Kramer and Sprenger.

The Church itself had little to offer the suffering peasantry:

On Sundays, after Mass, the sick came in scores, crying for help, — and words were all they got: "You have sinned, and God is afflicting you. Thank him; you will suffer so much the less torment in the life to come. Endure, suffer, die. Has not the Church its prayers for the dead?"

(Jules Michelet, *Satanism and Witchcraft*)

When faced with the misery of the poor, the Church turned to the dogma that experience in this world is fleeting and unimportant. But there was a double standard at work, for the Church was not against medical care for the upper class. Kings and nobles had their court physicians who were men, sometimes even priests. The real issue was control: Male upper class healing under the auspices of the Church was acceptable, female healing as part of a peasant subculture was not.

The Church saw its attack on peasant healers as an attack on *magic*, not medicine. The devil was believed to have real power on earth, and the use of that power by peasant women — whether for good or evil — was frightening to the Church and State. The greater their satanic powers to help themselves, the less they were dependent on God and the Church and the more they were potentially able to use their powers against God's order. Magic charms were thought to be at least as effective as prayer in healing the sick, but prayer was Church-sanctioned and controlled while incantations and charms were not. Thus magic cures, even when successful, were an accursed interference with the will of God, achieved with the help of the devil, and the cure itself was evil. There was no problem in distinguishing God's cures from the devil's, for obviously the Lord would work through priests and doctors rather than through peasant women.

The wise woman, or witch, had a host of remedies which had been tested in years of use. Many of the herbal remedies developed by witches still have their place in modern pharmacology. They had pain-killers, digestive aids and anti-inflammatory agents. They used ergot for the pain of labor at a time when the Church held that pain in labor was the Lord's just punishment for Eve's original sin. Ergot derivatives are the principal drugs used today to hasten labor and aid in the recovery from childbirth. Belladonna — still used today as an anti-spasmodic — was used by the witch-healers to inhibit uterine contractions when miscarriage threatened. Digitalis, still an important drug in treating heart ailments, is said to have been discovered by an English witch. Undoubtedly many of the witches' other remedies were purely magical, and owed their effectiveness — if they had any — to their reputation.

The witch-healer's methods were as great a threat (to the Catholic Church, if not the Protestant) as her results, for the witch was an empiricist: She relied on her senses rather than on faith or doctrine, she believed in trial and error, cause and effect. Her attitude was not religiously passive, but actively inquiring. She trusted her ability to find ways to deal with disease, pregnancy and childbirth — whether through medications or charms. In short, her magic was the science of her time.

The Church, by contrast, was deeply anti-empirical. It discredited the value of the material world, and had a profound distrust of the senses. There was no point in looking for natural laws that govern physical phenomena, for the world is created anew by God in every instant. Kramer and Sprenger, in the *Malleus*, quote St. Augustine on the deceptiveness of the senses:

. . .Now the motive of the will is something perceived through the senses or the intellect, both of which are subject to the power of the devil. For St. Augustine says in Book 83: This evil, which is of the devil, creeps in by all the sensual approaches; he places himself in figures, he adapts himself to colors, he attaches himself to sounds, he lurks in angry and wrongful conversation, he abides in smells, he impregnates with flavours and fills with certain exhalations all the channels of the understanding.

The senses are the devil's playground, the arena into which he will try to lure men away from Faith and into the conceits of the intellect or the delusions of carnality.

In the persecution of the witch, the anti-empiricist and the misogynist, anti-sexual obsessions of the Church coincide: Empiricism and sexuality both represent a surrender to the senses, a betrayal of faith. The witch was a triple threat to the Church: She was a woman, and not ashamed of it. She appeared to be part of an organized underground of peasant women. And she was a healer whose practice was based in empirical study. In the face of the repressive fatalism of Christianity, she held out the hope of change in this world.

The Rise of the European Medical Profession

While witches practiced among the people, the ruling classes were cultivating their own breed of secular healers: the university-trained physicians. In the century that preceded the beginning of the "witch-craze"—the thirteenth century—European medicine became firmly established as a secular science and a *profession*. The medical profession was actively engaged in the elimination of female healers—their exclusion from the universities, for example—long before the witch-hunts began.

For eight long centuries, from the fifth to the thirteenth, the other-wordly, anti-medical stance of the Church had stood in the way of the development of medicine as a respectable profession. Then, in the 13th century, there was a revival of learning, touched off by contact with the Arab world. Medical schools appeared in

The humors: sanguine, melancholy, hot-tempered, sluggish

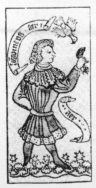 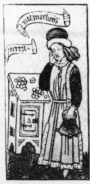 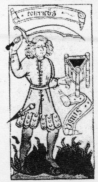 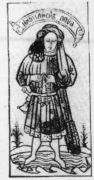

15

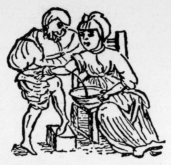

THE BENEFITS OF BLEEDING

the universities, and more and more young men of means sought medical training. The church imposed strict controls on the new profession, and allowed it to develop only within the terms set by Catholic doctrine. University-trained physicians were not permitted to practice without calling in a priest to aid and advise them, or to treat a patient who refused confession. By the fourteenth century their practice was in demand among the wealthy, as long as they continued to take pains to show that their attentions to the body did not jeopardize the soul. In fact, accounts of their medical training make it seem more likely that they jeopardized the *body*.

There was nothing in late medieval medical training that conflicted with church doctrine, and little that we would recognize as "science." Medical students, like other scholarly young gentlemen, spent years studying Plato, Aristotle and Christian theology. Their medical theory was largely restricted to the works of Galen, the ancient Roman physician who stressed the theory of "complexions" or "temperaments" of men, "wherefore the choleric are wrathful, the sanguine are kindly, the melancholy are envious," and so on. While a student, a doctor rarely saw any patients at all, and no experimentation of any kind was taught. Medicine was sharply differentiated from surgery, which was almost everywhere considered a degrading, menial craft, and the dissection of bodies was almost unheard of.

Confronted with a sick person, the university-trained physician had little to go on but superstition. Bleeding was a common practice, especially in the case of wounds. Leeches were applied according to the time, the hour, the air, and other similar considerations. Medical theories were often grounded more in "logic" than in observation: "Some foods brought on good humours, and others, evil humours. For example, nasturtium, mustard, and garlic produced reddish bile; lentils, cabbage and the meat of old goats and beeves begot black bile." Incantations, and quasi-religious rituals were thought to be effective: The physician to Edward II, who held a bachelor's degree in theology and a doctorate in medicine from Oxford, prescribed for toothache writing on the jaws of the patient, "In the name of the Father, the Son, and the Holy Ghost, Amen,", or touching a needle to a caterpillar and then to the tooth. A frequent treatment for leprosy was a broth made of the flesh of a black snake caught in a dry land among stones.

Such was the state of medical "science" at the time when witch-healers were persecuted for being practitioners of "magic". It was witches who developed an extensive understanding of bones and muscles, herbs and drugs, while physicians were still deriving their prognoses from astrology and alchemists were trying to turn lead into gold. So great was the witches' knowledge that in 1527, Paracelsus, considered the "father of modern medicine," burned his text on pharmaceuticals, confessing that he "had learned from the Sorceress all he knew."

The Suppression of Women Healers

The establishment of medicine as a profession, requiring university training, made it easy to bar women legally from practice. With few exceptions, the universities were closed to women (even to upper class women who could afford them), and licensing laws were established to prohibit all but university-trained doctors from practice. It was impossible to enforce the licensing laws consistently since there was only a handful of university-trained doctors compared to the great mass of lay healers. But the laws *could* be used selectively. Their first target was not the peasant healer, but the better off, literate woman healer who

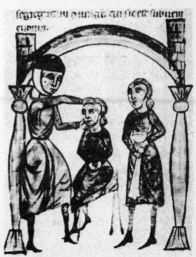

Woman treating dislocated jaw

competed for the same urban clientele as that of the university-trained doctors.

Take, for example, the case of Jacoba Felicie, brought to trial in 1322 by the Faculty of Medicine at the University of Paris, on charges of illegal practice. Jacoba was literate and had received some unspecified "special training" in medicine. That her patients were well off is evident from the fact that (as they testified in court) they had consulted well-known university-trained physicians before turning to her. The primary accusations brought against her were that

> . . .she would cure her patient of internal illness and wounds or of external abscesses. She would visit the sick assiduously and continue to examine the urine in the manner of physicians, feel the pulse, and touch the body and limbs.

Six witnesses affirmed that Jacoba had cured them, even after numerous doctors had given up, and one patient declared that she was wiser in the art of surgery and medicine than any master physician or surgeon in Paris. But these testimonials were used

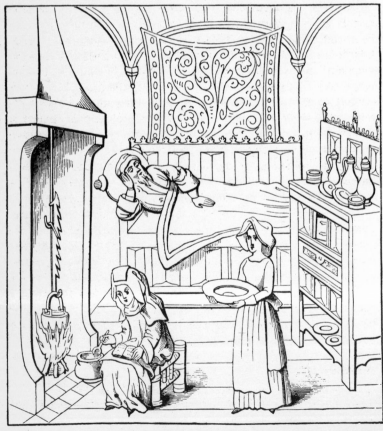

THE LADY AS PHYSICIAN.

against her, for the charge was not that she was incompetent, but that—as a woman—she dared to cure at all.

Along the same lines, English physicians sent a petition to Parliament bewailing the "worthless and presumptuous women who usurped the profession" and asking the imposition of fines and "long imprisonment" on any woman who attempted to "use the practyse of Fisyk." By the 14th century, the medical profession's campaign against urban, educated women healers was virtually complete throughout Europe. Male doctors had won a clear monopoly over the practice of medicine among the upper classes (except for obstetrics, which remained the province of female midwives even among the upper classes for another three centuries.) They were ready to take on a key role in the elimination of the great mass of female healers—the "witches."

The partnership between Church, State and medical profession reached full bloom in the witch trials. The doctor was held up the medical "expert," giving an aura of science to the whole proceeding. He was asked to make judgments about whether certain women were witches and whether certain afflictions had been caused by witchcraft. The *Malleus* says: "And if it is asked how it is possible to distinguish whether an illness is caused by witchcraft or by some natural physical defect, we answer that the first [way] is by means of the *judgement of doctors...*" [Emphasis added]. In the witch-hunts, the Church explicitly legitimized the doctors' professionalism, denouncing non-professional healing as equivalent to heresy: "If a woman dare to cure *without having studied* she is a witch and must die." (Of course, there wasn't any way for a woman to study.) Finally, the witch craze provided a handy excuse for the doctor's failings in everyday practice: Anything he couldn't cure was obviously the result of sorcery.

The distinction between "female" superstition and "male" medicine was made final by the very roles of the doctor and the witch at the trial. The trial in one stroke established the male physician on a moral and intellectual plane vastly above the female healer he was called to judge. It placed him on the side of God and Law, a professional on par with lawyers and theologians, while it placed her on the side of darkness, evil and magic. He owed his new status not to medical or scientific achievements of his own, but to the Church and State he served so well.

The Aftermath

Witch hunts did not eliminate the lower class woman healer, but they branded her forever as superstitious and possibly malevolent.

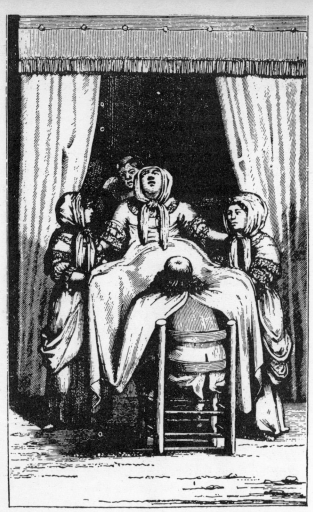

Doctor delivering under a sheet, for modesty's sake

So thoroughly was she discredited among the emerging middle classes that in the 17th and 18th centuries it was possible for male practitioners to make serious inroads into that last preserve of female healing—midwifery. Nonprofessional male practitioners— "barber-surgeons"—led the assault in England, claiming technical superiority on the basis of their use of the obstetrical forceps. (The forceps were legally classified as a surgical instrument, and women were legally barred from surgical practice.) In the hands of the barber surgeons, obstetrical practice among the middle class was quickly transformed from a neighborly service into a lucrative business, which real physicians entered in force in the 18th century. Female midwives in England organized and charged the male intruders with commercialism and dangerous misuse of the forceps. But it was too late—the women were easily put down as ignorant "old wives" clinging to the superstitions of the past.

Women and the Rise of the American Medical Profession

In the US the male takeover of healing roles started later than in England or France, but ultimately went much further. There is probably no industrialized country with a lower percentage of women doctors than the US today: England has 24 percent; Russia has 75 percent; the US has only seven percent. And while midwifery—*female* midwifery—is still a thriving occupation in Scandinavia, the United Kingdom, the Netherlands, etc., it has been virtually outlawed here since the early twentieth century. By the turn of the century, medicine here was closed to all but a tiny minority of necessarily tough and well-heeled women. What was left was nursing, and this was in no way a substitute for the autonomous roles women had enjoyed as midwives and general healers.

The question is not so much how women got "left out" of medicine and left with nursing, but how did these categories arise at all? To put it another way: How did one particular set of healers, who happened to be male, white and middle class, manage to oust all the competing folk healers, midwives and other practitioners who had dominated the American medical scene in the early 1800's?

The conventional answer given by medical historians is, of course, that there always was one *true* American medical profession—a small band of men whose scientific and moral authority flowed in an unbroken stream from Hippocrates, Galen and the great European medical scholars. In frontier America these doctors had to combat, not only the routine problems of sickness and death, but the abuses of a host of lay practitioners—usually depicted as women, ex-slaves, Indians and drunken patent medicine salesmen. Fortunately for the medical profession, in the late 19th century the American public suddenly developed a healthy respect for the doctors' scientific knowledge, outgrew its earlier faith in quacks, and granted the true medical profession a lasting monopoly of the healing arts.

But the real answer is not in this made-up drama of science versus ignorance and superstition. It's part of the 19th century's long story of class and sex struggles for power in all areas of life.

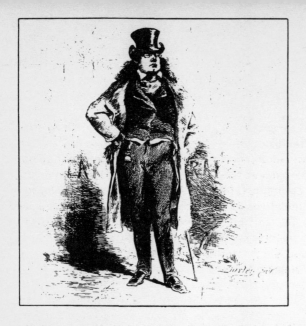

When women had a place in medicine, it was in a *people's* medicine. When that people's medicine was destroyed, there was no place for women—except in the subservient role of nurses. The set of healers who became *the* medical profession was distinguished not so much by its associations with modern science as by its associations with the emerging American business establishment. With all due respect to Pasteur, Koch and the other great European medical researchers of the 19th century, it was the Carnegies and Rockefellers who intervened to secure the final victory of the American medical profession.

The US in 1800 could hardly have been a more unpromising environment for the development of a medical profession, or any profession, for that matter. Few formally trained physicians had emigrated here from Europe. There were very few schools of medicine in America and very few institutions of higher learning altogether. The general public, fresh from a war of national liberation, was hostile to professionalism and "foreign" elitisms of any type.

In Western Europe, university-trained physicians already had a centuries' old monopoly over the right to heal. But in America, medical practice was traditionally open to anyone who could demonstrate healing skills—regardless of formal training, race or sex. Ann Hutchinson, the dissenting religious leader of the 1600's, was a practitioner of "general physik," as were many other ministers and their wives. The medical historian Joseph Kett reports that "one of the most respected medical men in late 18th century Windsor, Connecticut, for example, was a freed Negro called "Dr. Primus." In New Jersey, medical practice, except in extraordinary cases, was mainly in the hands of women as late as 1818..."

Women frequently went into joint practices with their husbands: The husband handling the surgery, the wife the midwifery and gynecology, and everything else shared. Or a woman might go into practice after developing skills through caring for family members or through an apprenticeship with a relative or other established healer. For example, Harriet Hunt, one of America's first trained female doctors, became interested in medicine during her sister's illness, worked for a while with a husband-wife "doctor" team, then simply hung out her own shingle. (Only later did she undertake formal training.)

Enter the Doctor

In the early 1800's there was also a growing number of formally trained doctors who took great pains to distinguish themselves from the host of lay practitioners. The most important real distinction was that the formally trained, or "regular" doctors as they called themselves, were male, usually middle class, and almost always more expensive than the lay competition. The "regulars'" practices were largely confined to middle and upper class people who could afford the prestige of being treated by a "gentleman" of their own class. By 1800, fashion even dictated that upper and middle class women employ male "regular" doctors for obstetrical care — a custom which plainer people regarded as grossly indecent.

In terms of medical skills and theory, the so-called "regulars" had nothing to recommend them over the lay practitioners. Their "formal training" meant little even by European standards of the time: Medical programs varied in length from a few months to two years; many medical schools had no clinical facilities; high school diplomas were not required for admission to medical schools. Not that serious academic training would have helped much anyway — there was no body of medical science to be trained in. Instead, the "regulars" were taught to treat most ills by "heroic" measures: massive bleeding, huge doses of laxatives, calomel (a laxative containing mercury) and, later, opium. (The European medical profession had little better to offer at this time either.) There is no doubt that these "cures" were often either fatal or more injurious than the original disease. In the judgement of Oliver Wendell Holmes, Sr., himself a distinguished physician, if all the medicines used by the "regular" doctors in the US were thrown into the ocean, it would be so much the better for mankind and so much the worse for the fishes.

The lay practitioners were undoubtedly safer and more effective than the "regulars." They preferred mild herbal medications, dietary changes and hand-holding to heroic interventions. Maybe they didn't know any more than the "regulars," but at least they were less likely to do the patient harm. Left alone, they might well have displaced the "regular" doctors with even middle class consumers in time. But they didn't know the right people. The "regulars," with their close ties to the upper class, had legislative clout. By 1830, 13 states had passed medical licensing laws outlawing "irregular" practice and establishing the "regulars" as the only legal healers.

It was a premature move. There was no popular support for the idea of medical professionalism, much less for the particular set of healers who claimed it. And there was no way to enforce the new laws: The trusted healers of the common people could not be just legislated out of practice. Worse still—for the "regulars"—this early grab for medical monopoly inspired mass indignation in the form of a radical, popular health movement which came close to smashing medical elitism in America once and for all.

The Popular Health Movement

The Popular Health Movement of the 1830's and 40's is usually dismissed in conventional medical histories as the high-tide of quackery and medical cultism. In reality it was the medical front of a general social upheaval stirred up by feminist and working class movements. Women were the backbone of the Popular Health

"Regular" doctors try water treatment

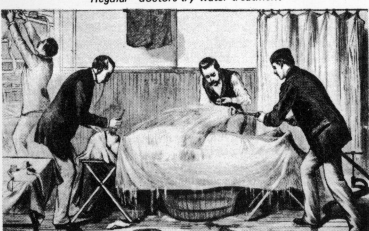

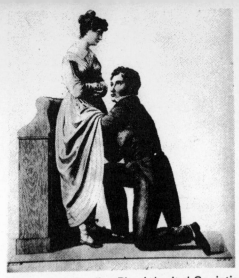

Gynecological exam

Movement. "Ladies Physiological Societies," the equivalent of our know-your-body courses, sprang up everywhere, bringing rapt audiences simple instruction in anatomy and personal hygiene. The emphasis was on preventive care, as opposed to the murderous "cures" practiced by the "regular" doctors. The Movement ran up the banner for frequent bathing (regarded as a vice by many "regular" doctors of the time), loose-fitting female clothing, whole grain cereals, temperance, and a host of other issues women could relate to. And, at about the time that Margaret Sanger's mother was a little girl, some elements of the Movement were already pushing birth control.

The Movement was a radical assault on medical elitism, and an affirmation of the traditional people's medicine. "Every man his own doctor," was the slogan of one wing of the Movement, and they made it very clear that they meant every woman too. The "regular," licensed, doctors were attacked as members of the "parasitic, non-producing classes," who survived only because of the upper class' "lurid taste" for calomel and bleeding. Universities (where the elite of the "regular" doctors were trained) were denounced as places where students "learn to look upon labor as servile and demeaning" and to identify with the upper class. Working class radicals rallied to the cause, linking "King-craft, Priest-craft, Lawyer-craft and Doctor-craft" as the four great evils of the time. In New York State, the Movement was represented in the legislature by a member of the Workingman's Party, who took every opportunity to assaiil the "privileged doctors."

The "regular" doctors quickly found themselves outnumbered and cornered. From the left-wing of the Popular Health Movement came a total rejection of "doctoring" as a paid occupation—much

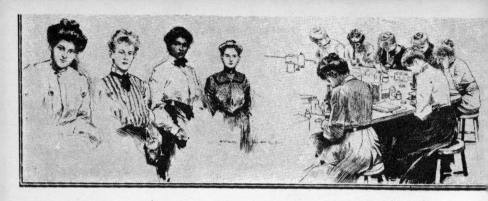

less as an overpaid "profession." From the moderate wing came a host of new medical philosophies, or sects, to compete with the "regulars" on their own terms: Eclecticism, Grahamism, Homeopathy, plus many minor ones. The new sects set up their own medical schools, (emphasizing preventive care and mild herbal cures), and started graduating their own doctors. In this context of medical ferment, the old "regulars" began to look like just another sect, a sect whose particular philosophy happened to lean towards calomel, bleeding and the other stand-by's of "heroic" medicine. It was impossible to tell who were the "real" doctors, and by the 1840's, medical licensing laws had been repealed in almost all of the states.

The peak of the Popular Health Movement coincided with the beginnings of an organized feminist movement, and the two were so closely linked that it's hard to tell where one began and the other left off. "This crusade for women's health [the Popular Health Movement] was related both in cause and effect to the demand for women's rights in general, and the health and feminist movements become indistinguishable at this point," according to Richard Shryock, the well-known medical historian. The health movement was concerned with women's rights in general, and the women's movement was particularly concerned with health and with women's access to medical training.

In fact, leaders of both groups used the prevailing sex stereotypes to argue that women were even better equipped to be doctors than men. "We cannot deny that women possess superior capacities for the science of medicine," wrote Samuel Thomson, a Health Movement leader, in 1834. (However, he felt surgery and the care of males should be reserved for male practitioners.) Feminists, like Sarah Hale, went further, exclaiming in 1852: "Talk about this [medicine] being the appropriate sphere for man and his alone! With tenfold more plausibility and reason we say it is the appropriate sphere for woman, and hers alone."

The new medical sects' schools did, in fact, open their doors to women at a time when "regular" medical training was all but closed to them. For example, Harriet Hunt was denied admission to Harvard Medical College, and instead went to a sectarian school for her formal training. (Actually, the Harvard faculty had voted to admit her—along with some black male students— but the students threatened to riot if they came.) The "regular" physicians could take the credit for training Elizabeth Blackwell, America's first female "regular," but her alma mater (a small school in upstate New York) quickly passed a resolution barring further female students. The first generally co-ed medical school was the "irregular" Eclectic Central Medical College of New York, in Syracuse. Finally, the first two all-female medical colleges, one in Boston and one in Philadelphia, were themselves "irregular."

Feminist researchers should really find out more about the Popular Health Movement. From the perspective of our movement today, it's probably more relevant than the women's suffrage struggle. To us, the most tantalizing aspects of the Movement are: (1) That it represented both class struggle and feminist struggle: Today, it's stylish in some quarters to write off purely feminist issues as middle class concerns. But in the Popular Health Movement we see a coming together of feminist and working class energies. Is this because the Popular Health Movement naturally attracted dissidents of all kinds, or was there some deeper identity of purpose? (2) The Popular Health Movement was not just a movement for more and better medical care, but for a radically different kind of health care: It was a substantive challenge to the prevailing medical dogma, practice and theory. Today we tend to confine our critiques to the organization of medical care, and assume that the scientific substratum of medicine is unassailable. We too should be developing the capability for the critical study of medical "science"—at least as it relates to women.

Doctors on the Offensive

At its height in the 1830's and 1840's, the Popular Health Movement had the "regular" doctors—the professional ancestors of today's physicians—running scared. Later in the 19th century, as the grassroots energy ebbed and the Movement degenerated into a set of competing sects, the "regulars" went back on the offensive. In 1848, they pulled together their first national organization, pretentiously named *the American* Medical Association (AMA.) County and state medical societies, many of which had practically disbanded during the height of medical anarchy in the '30s and '40s, began to reform.

Throughout the latter part of the 19th century, the "regulars" relentlessly attacked lay practitioners, sectarian doctors and women practitioners in general. The attacks were linked: Women practitioners could be attacked because of their sectarian leanings; sects could be attacked because of their openness to women. The arguments against women doctors ranged from the paternalistic (how could a respectable woman travel at night to a medical emergency?) to the hardcore sexist. In his presidential address to the AMA in 1871, Dr. Alfred Stille, said:

> Certain women seek to rival men in manly sports...and the strongminded ape them in all things, even in dress. In doing so they may command a sort of admiration such as all monstrous productions inspire, especially when they aim towards a higher type than their own.

The virulence of the American sexist opposition to women in medicine has no parallel in Europe. This is probably because: First, fewer European women were aspiring to medical careers at this time. Second, feminist movements were nowhere as strong as in the U S , and here the male doctors rightly associated the entrance of women into medicine with organized feminism. And, third, the European medical profession was already more firmly established and hence less afraid of competition.

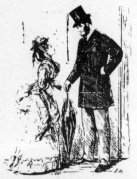

THE COMING RACE
Doctor Evangeline. 'BY THE BYE, MR SAWYER, ARE YOU ENGAGED TOMORROW AFTERNOON? I HAVE RATHER A TICKLISH OPERATION TO PERFORM—AN AMPUTATION, YOU KNOW.'
Mr Sawyer. 'I SHALL BE VERY HAPPY TO DO IT FOR YOU.'
Dr Evangeline. 'O, NO, NOT *THAT*! BUT WILL YOU KINDLY COME AND ADMINISTER THE CHLOROFORM FOR ME?' *14.9.1872*

The rare woman who did make it into a "regular" medical school faced one sexist hurdle after another. First there was the continuous harassment—often lewd—by the male students. There were professors who wouldn't discuss anatomy with a lady present. There were textbooks like a well-known 1848 obstetrical text which stated, "She [Woman] has a head almost too small for intellect but just big enough for love." There were respectable gynecological theories of the injurious effects of intellectual activity on the female reproductive organs.

Having completed her academic work, the would-be woman doctor usually found the next steps blocked. Hospitals were usually closed to women doctors, and even if they weren't, the internships were not open to women. If she did finally make it into practice, she found her brother "regulars" unwilling to refer patients to her and absolutely opposed to her membership in their medical societies.

And so it is all the stranger to us, and all the sadder, that what we might call the "women's health movement" began, in the late 19th century, to dissociate itself from its Popular Health Movement past and to strive for respectability. Members of irregular sects were purged from the faculties of the women's medical colleges. Female medical leaders such as Elizabeth Blackwell joined male "regulars" in demanding an end to lay midwifery and "a complete medical education" for all who practiced obstetrics. All this at a time when the "regulars" still had little or no "scientific" advantage over the sect doctors or lay healers.

The explanation, we suppose, was that the women who were

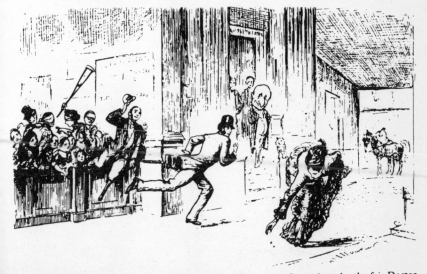

32. Dr. Meilanion Jones, finding himself outstripped in the race for patients by the fair Doctoress Atalanta Robinson, gallantly throws her a wedding ring and wins the day.

likely to seek formal medical training at this time were middle class. They must have found it easier to identify with the middle class "regular" doctors than with lower class women healers or with the sectarian medical groups (which had earlier been identified with radical movements.) The shift in allegiance was probably made all the easier by the fact that, in the cities, female lay practitioners were increasingly likely to be immigrants. (At the same time, the possibilities for a cross-class women's movement on *any* issue were vanishing as working class women went into the factories and middle class women settled into Victorian ladyhood.) Whatever the exact explanation, the result was that middle class women had given up the substantive attack on male medicine, and accepted the terms set by the emerging male medical profession.

Professional Victory

The "regulars" were still in no condition to make another bid for medical monopoly. For one thing, they still couldn't claim to have any uniquely effective methods or special body of knowledge. Besides, an occupational group doesn't gain a professional monopoly on the basis of technical superiority alone. A recognized profession is not just a group of self-proclaimed experts; it is a group which has authority *in the law* to select its own members and regulate their practice, i.e., to monopolize a certain field without outside interference. How does a particular group gain full professional status? In the words of sociologist Elliot Freidson:

A profession attains and maintains its position by virtue of the protection and patronage of some elite segment of society which has been persuaded that there is some special value in its work.

In other words, professions are the creation of a ruling class. To become *the* medical profession, the "regular" doctors needed, above all, ruling class patronage.

By a lucky coincidence for the "regulars," both the science and the patronage became available around the same time, at the turn of the century. French and especially German scientists brought forth the germ theory of disease which provided, for the first time in human history, a rational basis for disease prevention and therapy. While the run-of-the-mill American doctor was still mumbling about "humors" and dosing people with calomel, a tiny medical elite was travelling to German universities to learn the new science. They returned to the US filled with reformist zeal. In 1893 German-trained doctors (funded by local philanthropists) set up the first American German-style medical school, Johns Hopkins.

As far as curriculum was concerned, the big innovation at Hopkins was integrating lab work in basic science with expanded clinical training. Other reforms included hiring full time faculty, emphasizing research, and closely associating the medical school with a full university. Johns Hopkins also introduced the modern pattern of medical education——four years of medical school following four years of college—which of course barred most working class and poor people from the possibility of a medical education.

Meanwhile the US was emerging as the industrial leader of the world. Fortunes built on oil, coal and the ruthless exploitation of American workers were maturing into financial empires. For the first time in American history, there were sufficient concentrations of corporate wealth to allow for massive, organized philanthropy, i.e., organized ruling class intervention in the social, cultural and political life of the nation. Foundations were created as the lasting instruments of this intervention—the Rockefeller and Carnegie foundations appeared in the first decade of the 20th century. One of the earliest and highest items on their agenda was medical "reform," the creation of a respectable, scientific American medical profession.

The group of American medical practitioners that the foundations chose to put their money behind was, naturally enough, the scientific elite of the "regular" doctors. (Many of these men were themselves ruling class, and all were urbane, university-trained gentlemen.) Starting in 1903, foundation money began to pour into medical schools by the millions. The conditions were

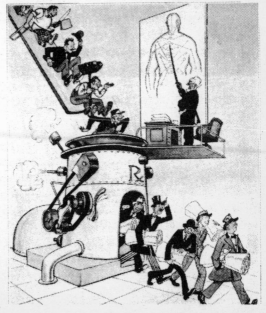

Medical diploma mill

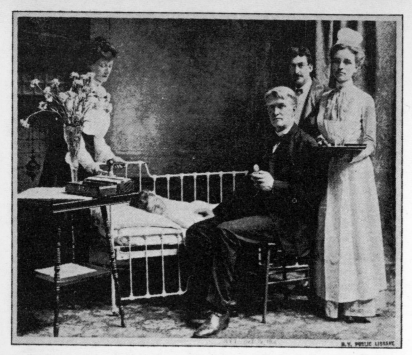

clear: Conform to the Johns Hopkins model or close. To get the message across, the Carnegie Corporation sent a staff man, Abraham Flexner, out on a national tour of medical schools—from Harvard right down to the last third-rate commercial schools.

Flexner almost singlehandedly decided which schools would get the money—and hence survive. For the bigger and better schools (i.e, those which already had enough money to begin to institute the prescribed reforms), there was the promise of fat foundation grants. Harvard was one of the lucky winners, and its president could say smugly in 1907, ''Gentlemen, the way to get endowments for medicine is to improve medical education.'' As for the smaller, poorer schools, which included most of the sectarian schools and special schools for blacks and women—Flexner did not consider them worth saving. Their options were to close, or to remain open and face public denunciation in the report Flexner was preparing.

The Flexner Report, published in 1910, was the foundations' ultimatum to American medicine. In its wake, medical schools closed by the score, including six of America's eight black medical schools and the majority of the ''irregular'' schools which had been a haven for female students. Medicine was established once and for all as a branch of ''higher'' learning, accessible only through lengthy and expensive university training. It's certainly true that as medical knowledge grew, lengthier training did become necessary. But Flexner and the foundations had no intention of making such training available to the great mass of lay healers and "irregular" doctors. Instead, doors were slammed shut to blacks, to the majority of women and to poor white men. (Flexner in his report bewailed the fact that any "crude boy or jaded clerk" had been able to seek medical training.) Medicine had become a white, male, middle class occupation

But it was more than an occupation. It had become, at last, a profession. To be more precise, one particular group of healers, the "regular" doctors, was now *the* medical profession. Their victory was not based on any skills of their own: The run-of-the-mill "regular" doctor did not suddenly acquire a knowledge of medical science with the publication of the Flexner report. But he did acquire the *mystique* of science. So what if his own alma mater had been condemned in the Flexner report; wasn't he a member of the AMA, and wasn't it in the forefront of scientific reform? The doctor had become—thanks to some foreign scientists and eastern foundations—the "man of science": beyond criticism, beyond regulation, very nearly beyond competition.

Outlawing the Midwives

In state after state, new, tough, licensing laws sealed the doctor's monopoly on medical practice. All that was left was to drive out the last holdouts of the old people's medicine—the midwives. In 1910, about 50 percent of all babies were delivered by midwives—most were blacks or working class immigrants. It was an intolerable situation to the newly emerging obstetrical specialty: For one thing, every poor woman who went to a midwife was one more case lost to academic teaching and research. America's vast lower class resources of obstetrical "teaching material" were being

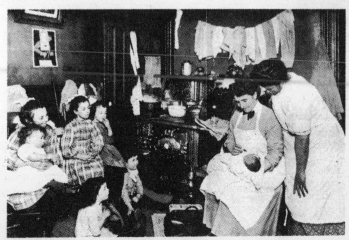

wasted on ignorant midwives. Besides which, poor women were spending an estimated $5 million a year on midwives—$5 million which could have been going to "professionals."

Publicly, however, the obstetricians launched their attacks on midwives in the name of science and reform. Midwives were ridiculed as "hopelessly dirty, ignorant and incompetent." Specifically, they were held responsible for the prevalence of puerperal sepsis (uterine infections) and neonatal ophthalmia (blindness due to parental infection with gonorrhea). Both conditions were easily preventable by techniques well within the grasp of the least literate midwife (hand-washing for puerperal sepsis, and eye drops for the ophthalmia.) So the obvious solution for a truly public-spirited obstetrical profession would have been to make the appropriate preventive techniques known and available to the mass of midwives. This is in fact what happened in England, Germany and most other European nations: Midwifery was upgraded through training to become an established, independent occupation.

But the American obstetricians had no real commitment to improved obstetrical care. In fact, a study by Johns Hopkins professor in 1912 indicated that most American doctors were *less* competent than the midwives. Not only were the doctors themselves unreliable about preventing sepsis and ophthalmia but they also tended to be too ready to use surgical techniques which endangered mother or child. If anyone, then, deserved a legal monopoly on obstetrical care, it was the midwives, not the MD's. But the doctors had power, the midwives didn't. Under intense pressure from the medical profession, state after state passed laws outlawing midwifery and restricting the practice of obstetrics to doctors. For poor and working class women, this actually meant worse—or no—obstetrical care. (For instance, a study of infant mortality rates in Washington showed an increase in infant mortality in the years immediately following the passage of the law forbidding midwifery.) For the new, male medical profession, the ban on midwives meant one less source of competition. Women had been routed from their last foothold as independent practitioners.

The Lady with the Lamp

The only remaining occupation for women in health was nursing. Nursing had not always existed as a paid occupation—it had to be invented. In the early 19th century, a "nurse" was simply a woman who happened to be nursing someone — a sick child or an aging relative. There were hospitals, and they did employ nurses. But the hospitals of the time served largely as refuges for the dying poor, with only token care provided. Hospital nurses, history has it, were a disreputable lot, prone to drunkenness, prostitution and thievery. And conditions in the hospitals were often scandalous. In the late 1870's a committee investigating New York's Bellevue Hopital could not find a bar of soap on the premises.

If nursing was not exactly an attractive field to women workers, it was a wide open arena for women *reformers*. To reform hospital care, you had to reform nursing, and to make nursing acceptable to doctors and to women of "good character," it had to be given a completely new image. Florence Nightingale got her change in the battle-front hospitals of the Crimean War, where she replaced the old camp-follower "nurses" with a bevy of disciplined, sober, middle-aged ladies. Dorothea Dix, an American hospital reformer, introduced the new breed of nurses in the Union hospitals of the Civil War.

The new nurse — "the lady with the lamp," selflessly tending the wounded — caught the popular imagination. Real nursing schools began to appear in England right after the Crimean War, and in the US right after the Civil War. At the same time, the number of hospitals began to increase to keep pace with the needs of medical education. Medical students needed hospitals to train in; good hospitals, as the doctors were learning, needed good nurses.

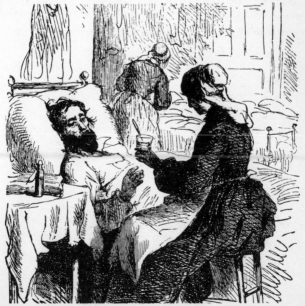

In fact, the first American nursing schools did their best to recruit actual upper class women as students. Miss Euphemia Van Rensselear, of an old aristocratic New York family, graced Bellevue's first class. And at Johns Hopkins, where Isabel Hampton trained nurses in the University Hospital, a leading doctor could only complain that:

> Miss Hampton has been most successful in getting probationers [students] of the upper class; but unfortunately, she selects them altogether for their good looks and the House staff is by this time in a sad state.

Let us look a little more closely at the women who invented nursing, because, in a very real sense, nursing as we know it today is the product of their oppression as upper class Victorian women. Dorothea Dix was an heiress of substantial means. Florence Nightingale and Louisa Schuyler (the moving force behind the creation of America's first Nightingale-style nursing school) were genuine aristocrats. They were refugees from the enforced leisure of Victorian ladyhood. Dix and Nightingale did not begin to carve out their reform careers until they were in their thirties, and faced with the prospect of a long, useless spinsterhood. They focused their energies on the care of the sick because this was a "natural" and acceptable interest for ladies of their class.

Nightingale and her immediate disciples left nursing with the indelible stamp of their own class biases. Training emphasized character, not skills. The finished products, the Nightingale nurse, was simply the ideal Lady, transplanted from home to the hospital, and absolved of reproductive responsibilities. To the doctor, she brought the wifely virtue of absolute obedience. To the patient, she

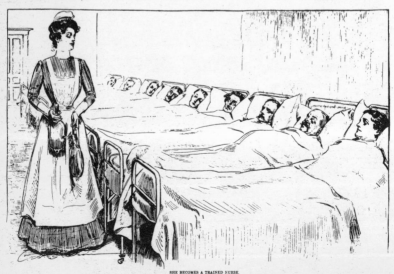

SHE BECOMES A TRAINED NURSE.

brought the selfless devotion of a mother. To the lower level hospital employees, she brought the firm but kindly discipline of a household manager accustomed to dealing with servants.

But, despite the glamorous "lady with the lamp" image, most of nursing work was just low-paid, heavy-duty housework. Before long, most nursing schools were attracting only women from working class and lower middle class homes, whose only other options were factory or clerical work. But the philosophy of nursing education did not change — after all, the educators were still middle and upper class women. If anything, they toughened their insistence on lady-like character development, and the socialization of nurses became what it has been for most of the 20th century: the imposition of upper class cultural values on working class women. (For example, until recently, most nursing students were taught such upper class graces as tea pouring, art appreciation, etc. Practical nurses are still taught to wear girdles, use make-up, and in general mimic the behavior of a "better" class of women.)

But the Nightingale nurse was not just the projection of upper class ladyhood onto the working world: She embodied the very spirit of femininity as defined by sexist Victorian society — she was Woman. The inventors of nursing saw it as a natural vocation for women, second only to motherhood. When a group of English nurses proposed that nursing model itself after the medical profession, with exams and licensing, Nightingale responded that "...nurses cannot be registered and examined *any more than mothers.*"[Emphasis added.] Or, as one historian of nursing put it,

nearly a century later, "Woman is an instinctive nurse, taught by

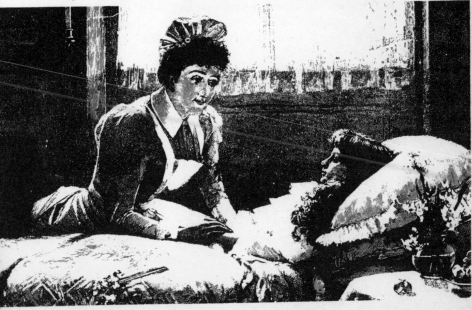

Mother Nature." (Victor Robinson, MD. *White Caps, The Story of Nursing*) If women were instinctive nurses, they were not, in the Nightingale view, instinctive doctors. She wrote of the few female physicians of her time: "They have only tried to be men, and they have succeeded only in being third-rate men." Indeed, as the number of nursing students rose in the late 19th century, the number of female medical students began to decline. Woman had found her place in the health system.

Just as the feminist movement had not opposed the rise of medical professionalism, it did not challenge nursing as an oppressive female role. In fact, feminists of the late 19th century were themselves beginning to celebrate the nurse/mother image of femininity. The American women's movement had given up the struggle for full sexual equality to focus exclusively on the vote, and to get it, they were ready to adopt the most sexist tenets of Victorian ideology: Women need the vote, they argued, not because they are human, but because they are Mothers. "Woman is the mother of the race," gushed Boston feminist Julia Ward Howe, "the guardian of its helpless infancy, its earliest teacher, its most zealous champion. Woman is also the homemaker, upon her devolve the details which bless and beautify family life." And so on in paeans too painful to quote.

The women's movement dropped its earlier emphasis on opening up the professions to women: Why foresake Motherhood for the petty pursuits of males? And of course the impetus to attack professionalism itself as inherently sexist and elitist was long since dead. Instead, they turned to professionalizing women's natural functions. Housework was glamorized in the new discipline of "domestic science." Motherhood was held out as a vocation requiring much the same preparation and skill as nursing or teaching.

So while some women were professionalizing women's domestic roles, others were "domesticizing" professional roles, like nursing, teaching and, later, social work. For the woman who chose to express her feminine drives outside of the home, these occupations were presented as simple extensions of women's "natural" domestic role. Conversely the woman who remained at home was encouraged to see herself as a kind of nurse, teacher and counsellor practicing within the limits of the family. And so the middle class feminists of the late 1800's dissolved away some of the harsher contradictions of sexism.

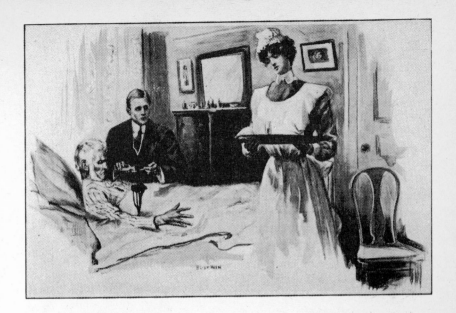

The Doctor Needs a Nurse

Of course, the women's movement was not in a position to decide on the future of nursing anyway. Only the medical profession was. At first, male doctors were a little skeptical about the new Nightingale nurses—perhaps suspecting that this was just one more feminine attempt to infiltrate medicine. But they were soon won over by the nurses' unflagging obedience. (Nightingale was a little obsessive on this point. When she arrived in the Crimea with her newly trained nurses, the doctors at first ignored them all. Nightingale refused to let her women lift a finger to help the thousands of sick and wounded soldiers until the doctors gave an order. Impressed, the doctors finally relented and set the nurses to cleaning up the hospital.) To the beleaguered doctors of the 19th century, nursing was a godsend: Here at last was a kind of health worker who did not want to compete with the "regulars," did not have a medical doctrine to push, and who seemed to have no other mission in life but to serve.

While the average regular doctor was making nurses welcome, the new scientific practitioners of the early 20th century were making them *necessary*. The new, post-Flexner physician, was even less likely than his predecessors to stand around and watch the progress of his "cures." He diagnosed, he prescribed, he moved on. He could not waste his talents, or his expensive academic training in the tedious details of bedside care. For this he needed a patient, obedient helper, someone who was not above the most menial tasks, in short, a nurse.

Healing, in its fullest sense, consists of both curing and caring, doctoring *and* nursing. The old lay healers of an earlier time had combined both functions, and were valued for both. (For example, midwives not only presided at the delivery, but lived in until the new mother was ready to resume care of her children.) But with the development of scientific medicine, and the modern medical profession, the two functions were split irrevocably. Curing became the exclusive province of the doctor; caring was relegated to the nurse. All credit for the patient's recovery went to the doctor and his "quick fix," for only the doctor participated in the mystique of Science. The nurse's activities, on the other hand, were barely distinguishable from those of a servant. She had no power, no magic, and no claim to the credit.

Doctoring and nursing arose as complementary functions, and the society which defined nursing as feminine could readily see doctoring as intrinsically "masculine." If the nurse was idealized Woman, the doctor was idealized Man—combining intellect and action, abstract theory and hard-headed pragmatism. The very qualities which fitted Woman for nursing barred her from doctoring, and vice versa. Her tenderness and innate spirituality were out of place in the harsh, linear world of science. His decisiveness and curiosity made him unfit for long hours of patient nurturing.

These sterotypes have proved to be almost unbreakable. Today's leaders of the American Nursing Association may insist that nursing is no longer a feminine vocation but a neuter

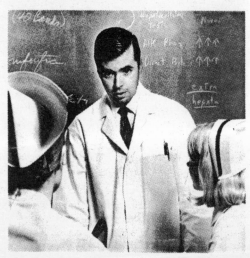

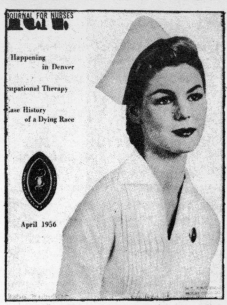

JOURNAL FOR NURSES

Happening
        in Denver

upational Therapy

ase History
        of a Dying Race

April 1956

"profession." They may call for more male nurses to change the "image," insist that nursing requires almost as much academic preparation as medicine, and so on. But the drive to "professionalize" nursing is, at best, a flight from the reality of sexism in the health system. At worst, it is sexist itself, deepening the division among women health workers and bolstering a heirarchy controlled by men.

Conclusion

We have our own moment of history to work out, our own struggles. What can we learn from the past that will help us—in a Women's Health Movement—today?
These are some of our conclusions:

☐ We have not been passive bystanders in the history of medicine. The present system was born in and shaped by the competition between male and female healers. The medical profession in particular is not just another institution which happens to discriminate against us: It is a fortress designed and erected to exclude us. This means to us that the sexism of the health system is not incidental, not just the reflection of the sexism of society in general or the sexism of individual doctors. It is historically older than medical science itself; it is deep-rooted, institutional sexism.
☐ Our enemy is not just "men" or their individual male

chauvinism: It is the whole class system which enabled male, upper class healers to win out and which forced us into subservience. Institutional sexism is sustained by a class system which supports male power.

☐ There is no historically consistent justification for the exclusion of women from healing roles. Witches were attacked for being pragmatic, empirical and immoral. But in the 19th century the rhetoric reversed: Women became too unscientific, delicate and sentimental. The *stereotypes* change to suit male convenience— *we* don't, and there is nothing in our "innate feminine nature" to justify our present subservience.

☐ Men maintain their power in the health system through their monopoly of scientific knowledge. We are mystified by science, taught to believe that it is hopelessly beyond our grasp. In our frustration, we are sometimes tempted to reject *science*, rather than to challenge the men who hoard it. But medical science could be a liberating force, giving us real control over our own bodies and power in our lives as health workers. At this point in our history, every effort to take hold of and share medical knowledge is a critical part of the struggle—know-your-body courses and literature, self-help projects, counselling, women's free clinics.

☐ Professionalism in medicine is nothing more than the institutionalization of a male upper class monopoly. We must never confuse professionalism with expertise. Expertise is something to work for and to share; professionalism is—by definition—elitist and exclusive, sexist, racist and classist. In the American past, women who sought formal medical training were too ready to accept the professionalism that went with it. They made *their* gains in status—but only on the backs of their less privileged sisters— midwives, nurses and lay healers. Our goal today should never be to open up the exclusive medical profession to women, but to open up medicine—to all women.

☐ This means that we must begin to break down the distinctions and barriers between women health workers and women consumers. We should build shared concerns: Consumers aware of women's needs as workers, workers in touch with women's needs as consumers. Women workers can play a leadership role in collective self-help and self-teaching projects, and in attacks on health institutions. But they need support and solidarity from a strong women's consumer movement.

☐ Our oppression as women health workers today is inextricably linked to our oppression as women. Nursing, our predominate role in the health system, is simply a workplace extension of our roles as wife and mother. The nurse is socialized to believe that rebellion violates not only her "professionalism," but her very femininity. This means that the male medical elite has a very special stake in the maintenance of sexism in the society at large: Doctors are the bosses in an industry where the workers are primarily women. Sexism in the society at large insures that the female majority of the health workforce are "good" workers—docile and passive. Take away sexism and you take away one of the mainstays of the health hierarchy.

What this means to us in practice is that in the health system there is no way to separate worker organizing from feminist organizing. To reach out to women health workers *as workers* is to reach out to them as *women*.

Bibliography

The Manufacture of Madness, by Thomas Szasz, M.D., Delta Books, 1971. Szasz asserts that institutional phychiatry is the modern version of the witch-hunts, with the patient in the role of the witch. We are indebted to him for first presenting witchcraft in the context of the struggle between professionals and lay healers. See especially the chapter on "The Witch as Healer."

Satanism and Witchcraft, by Jules Michelet. The Citadel Press, 1939. A mid-nineteenth century work by a famous French historian. A vivid book on the Middle Ages, superstition and the Church, with a discussion of "satan as physician."

The Malleus Maleficarum, by Heinrich Kramer and James Sprenger, translated by Rev. Montague Summers. The Pushkin Press, London, 1928. Difficult medieval writing, but by far the best source for the day-to-day operations of the witch-hunts, and for insights into the mentality of the witch-hunter.

The History of Witchcraft and Demonology, by Rev. Montague Summers. University Books, New York, 1956. Written in the 1920's by a Catholic priest and defender—really!—of the witch-hunts. Attacks the witch as "heretic," "anarchist," and "bawd."

Witchcraft, by Pennethrone Hughes. Penguin Books, 1952. A general introduction and survey.

Women Healers in Medieval Life and Literature, by Muriel Joy Hughes. Books for Libraries Press, Freeport, New York, 1943. A conservatively written book, with good information on the state of academic medicine and on women lay doctors and midwives. Unfortunately, it dismisses the whole question of witchcraft.

The Witch-Cult in Western Europe, by Margaret Alice Murray. Oxford University Press, 1921. Dr. Murray was the first person to present the anthropological view, now widely accepted, that witchcraft represented, in part, the survival among the people of a pre-Christian religion.

A Mirror of Witchcraft, by Christina Hole. Chatto and Windus, London, 1957. A source-book of extracts from trial reports and other writings, mostly from English witch trials of the 16th and 17th centuries.

The Formation of the American Medical Profession: The Role of Institutions, 1780-1860, by Joseph Kett. Yale University Press, 1968. Conservative point of view, but full of scattered information on lay healers. He discusses the politically radical nature of the Popular Health Movement in Chapter Four.

Medicine in America: Historical Essays, by Richard H. Shryock. Johns Hopkins Press, 1966. A readable, wide-ranging and fairly liberal book. See especially the chapters on "Women in American Medicine" and "The Popular Health Movement."

American Medicine and the Public Interest, by Rosemary Stevens. Yale University Press 1971. Long and dry, but useful for the early chapters on the formation of the American medical profession and the role of the foundations.

Medical Education in the US and Canada, by Abraham Flexner, Carnegie Foundation, 1910. (Available from University Microfilms,Ltd., Ann Arbor.) The famous "Flexner Report" that changed the face of American medical education. Some reasonable proposals, but amazing elitism, racism and sexism.

The History of Nursing, by Richard Shryock. N.B. Saunders, 1959. Better than most nursing histories — which are usually glorifications of nursing by nursing educators — but much worse than Shyrock's medical histories.

Lonely Crusader: The Life of Florence Nightingale, by Cecil Woodham-Smith. McGraw Hill, 1951. A richly detailed biography which puts nursing in the context of the oppression of upper class Victorian women.

Glances and Glimpses, by Harriet K. Hunt. Source Book Press, 1970. Rambling autobiography of a feminist and "irregular" woman doctor of the mid-19th century. It's useful for its descriptions of the state of medical practice at the time.

"The American Midwife Controversy: A Crisis of Professionalization," by Frances E. Kobrin. *Bulletin of the History of Medicine,* July-August 1966, p. 350. Restrained and scholarly account of the outlawing of American midwives. Very worthwhile reading.

The Feminist Press at The City University of New York offers alternatives in education and in literature. Founded in 1970, this nonprofit, tax-exempt educational and publishing organization works to eliminate stereotypes in books and schools and to provide literature with a broad vision of human potential. The publishing program includes reprints of important works by women, feminist biographies of women, multicultural anthologies, a cross-cultural memoir series, and nonsexist children's books. Curricular materials, bibliographies, directories, and a quarterly journal provide information and support for students and teachers of women's studies. Through publications and projects, The Feminist Press contributes to the rediscovery of the history of women and the emergence of a more humane society.

New and Forthcoming Books

Always a Sister: The Feminism of Lillian D. Wald. A biography by Doris Groshen Daniels. $12.95 paper.

A Rising Public Voice: Women in Politics Worldwide. Edited by Alida Brill. Foreword by Gertrude Mongella. $17.95 paper, $35.00 cloth.

The Answer/La Respuesta (Including a Selection of Poems), by Sor Juana Inés de la Cruz. Critical edition and translation by Electa Arenal and Amanda Powell. $12.95 paper, $35.00 cloth.

Black and White Sat Down Together: The Reminiscences of an NAACP Founder, by Mary White Ovington. Edited and with a foreword by Ralph E.Luker. Afterword by Carolyn E. Wedin. $19.95 cloth.

The Dragon and the Doctor, by Barbara Danish. $5.95 paper.

Japanese Women: New Feminist Perspectives on the Past, Present, and Future, edited by Kumiko Fujimura-Fanselow and Atsuko Kameda. $16.95 paper, $45.00 cloth.

Seeds 2: Supporting Women's Work around the World, edited by Ann Leonard. Introduction by Martha Chen. Afterwords by Mayra Buvinic, Misrak Elias, Rounaq Jahan, Caroline Moser, and Kathleen Staudt. $12.95 paper, $35.00 cloth.

Streets: A Memoir of the Lower East Side. By Bella Spewack. Introduction by Ruth Limmer. Afterword by Lois Elias. $19.95 cloth.

Women of Color and the Multicultural Curriculum: Transforming the College Classroom, edited by Liza Fiol-Matta and Mariam K. Chamberlain. $18.95 paper, $35.00 cloth.

Prices subject to change. Individuals: Send check or money order (in U.S. dollars drawn on a U.S. bank) to The Feminist Press at The City University of New York, 311 East 94th Street, New York, NY 10128. Please include $4.00 postage and handling for the first book, $1.00 for each additional. For VISA/MasterCard orders call (212) 360-5794. Bookstores, libraries, wholesalers: Feminist Press titles are distributed to the trade by Consortium Book Sales and Distribution, (800) 283-3572.